Bathtime!

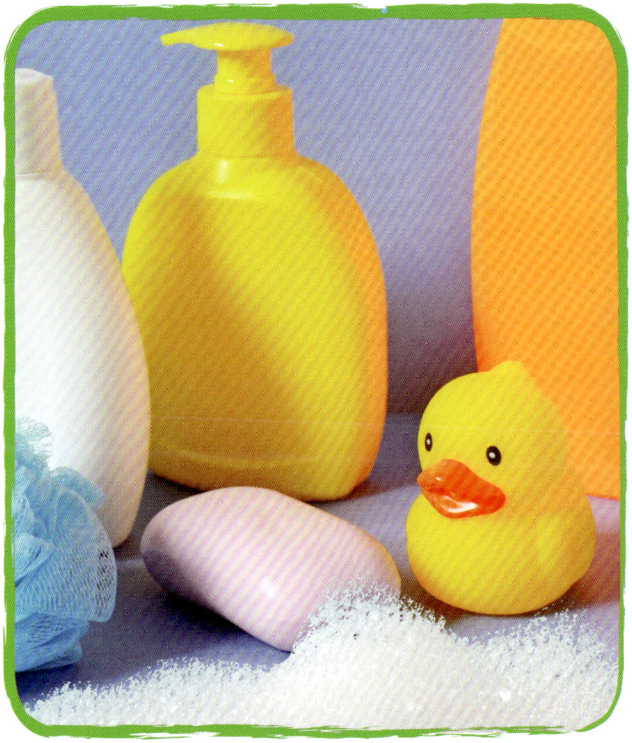

Dona Herweck Rice

Publishing Credits

Rachelle Cracchiolo, M.S.Ed., *Publisher*
Conni Medina, M.A.Ed., *Managing Editor*
Nika Fabienke, Ed.D., *Content Director*
Véronique Bos, *Creative Director*
Shaun N. Bernadou, *Art Director*
Valerie Morales, *Associate Editor*
John Leach, *Assistant Editor*
Courtney Roberson, *Senior Graphic Designer*

Image Credits: All images from iStock and/or Shutterstock.

Teacher Created Materials
5301 Oceanus Drive
Huntington Beach, CA 92649-1030
www.tcmpub.com

ISBN 978-1-4938-9839-8

Printed in China
51497

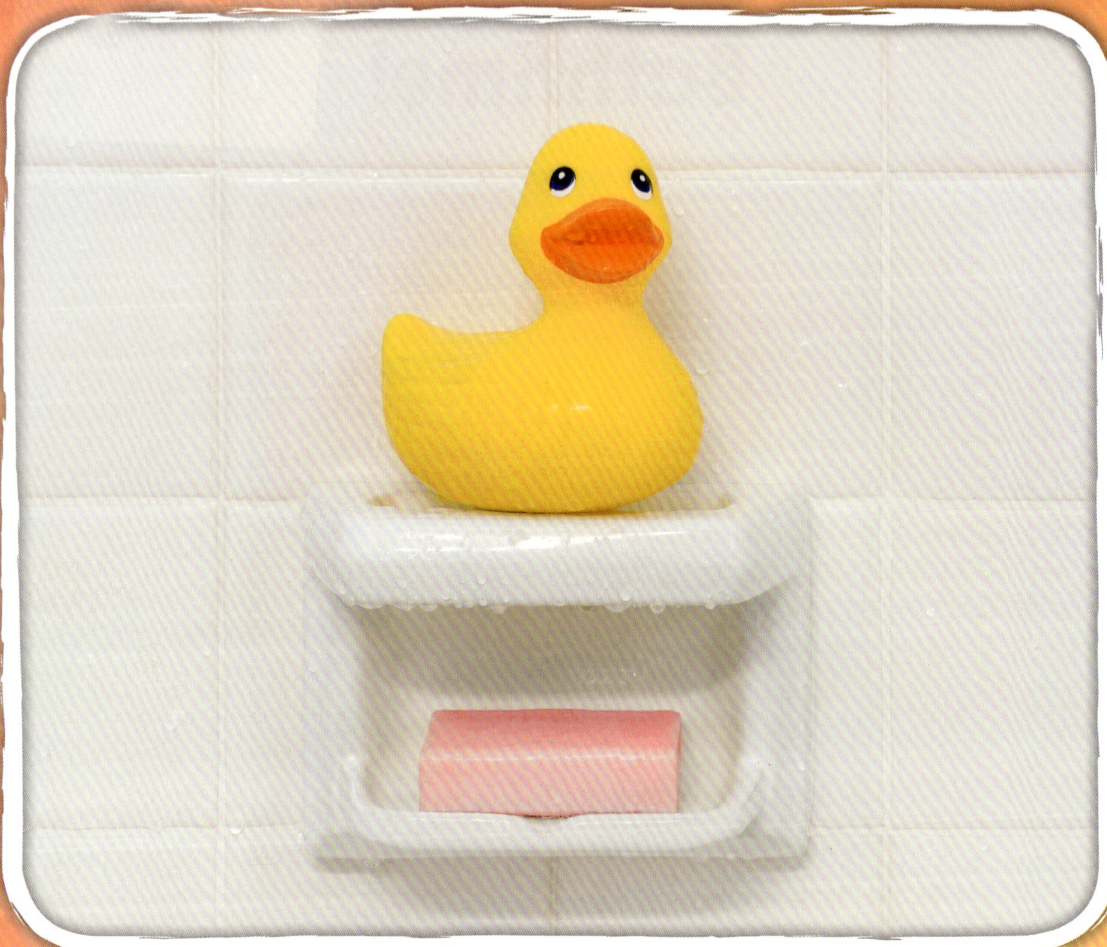

Go and find some

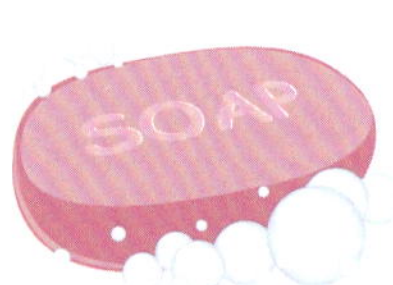

by the water.

soap

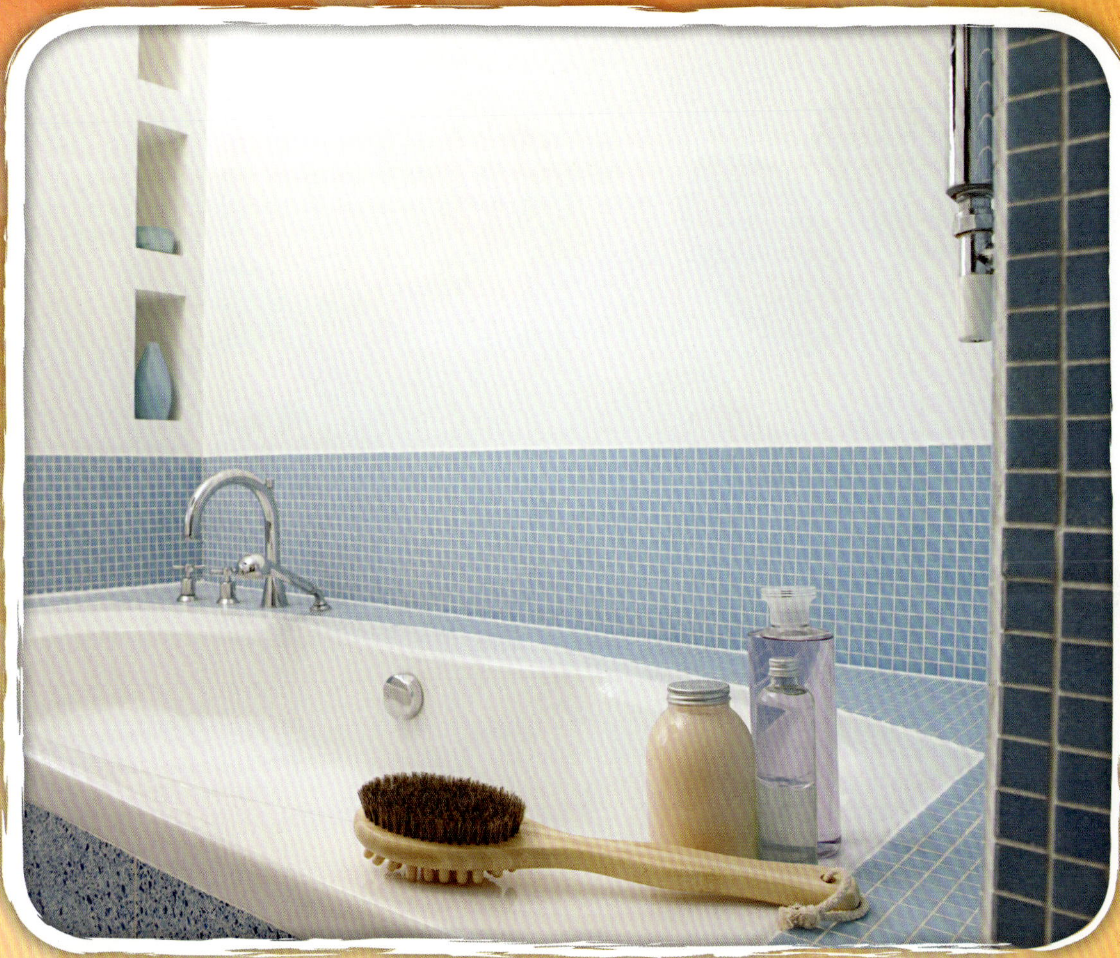

Go and find some

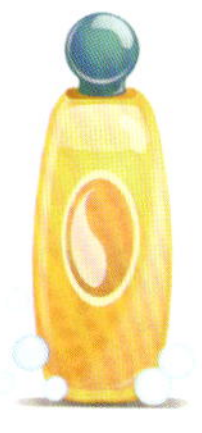

by the water.

bubble bath

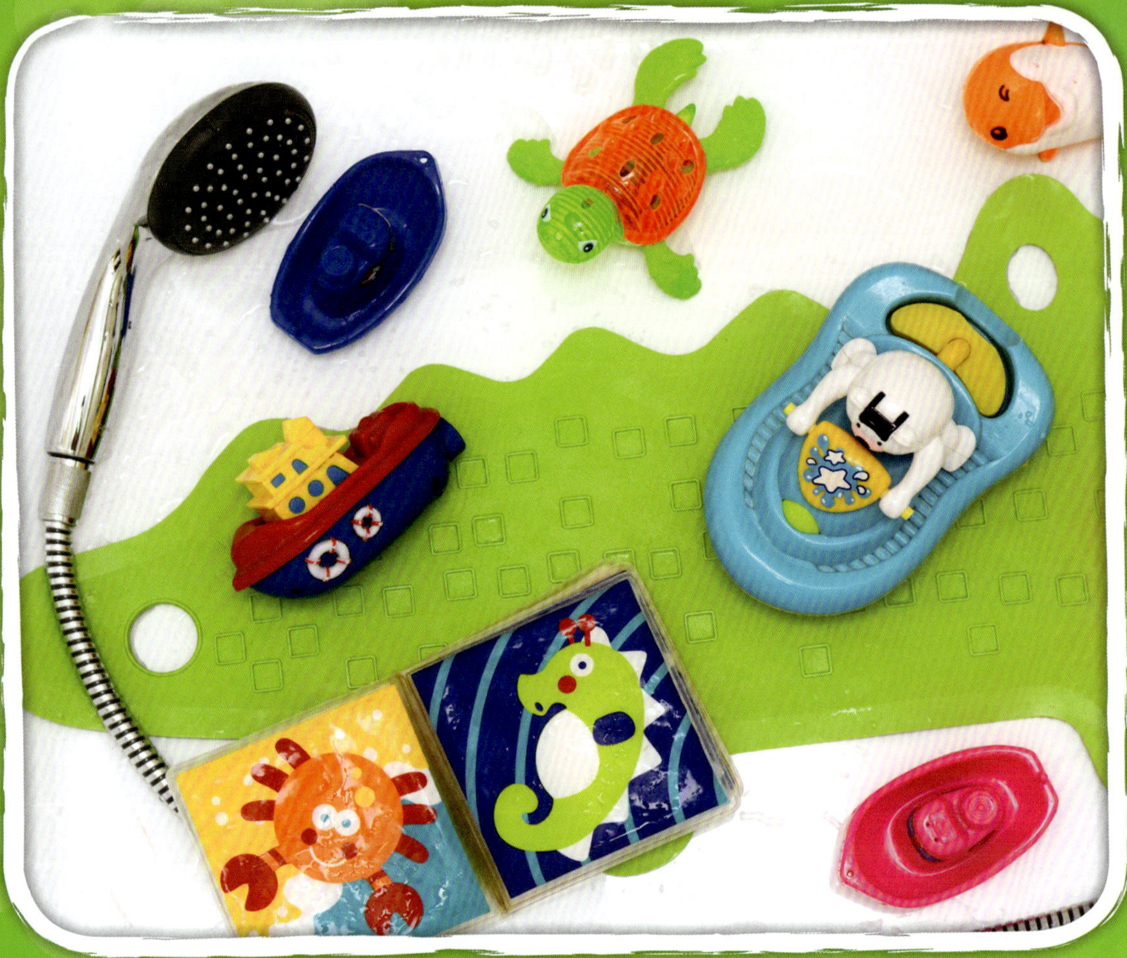

Go and find some

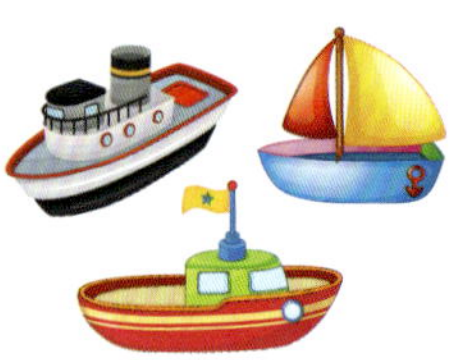 by the water.

boats

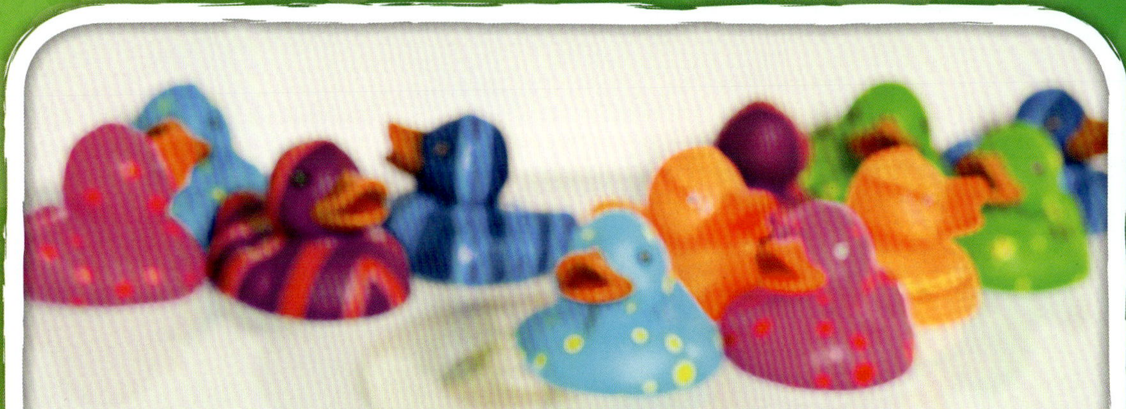

Go and find some

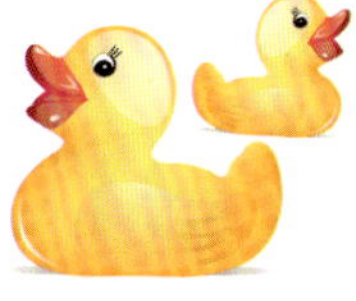 by the water.

rubber ducks

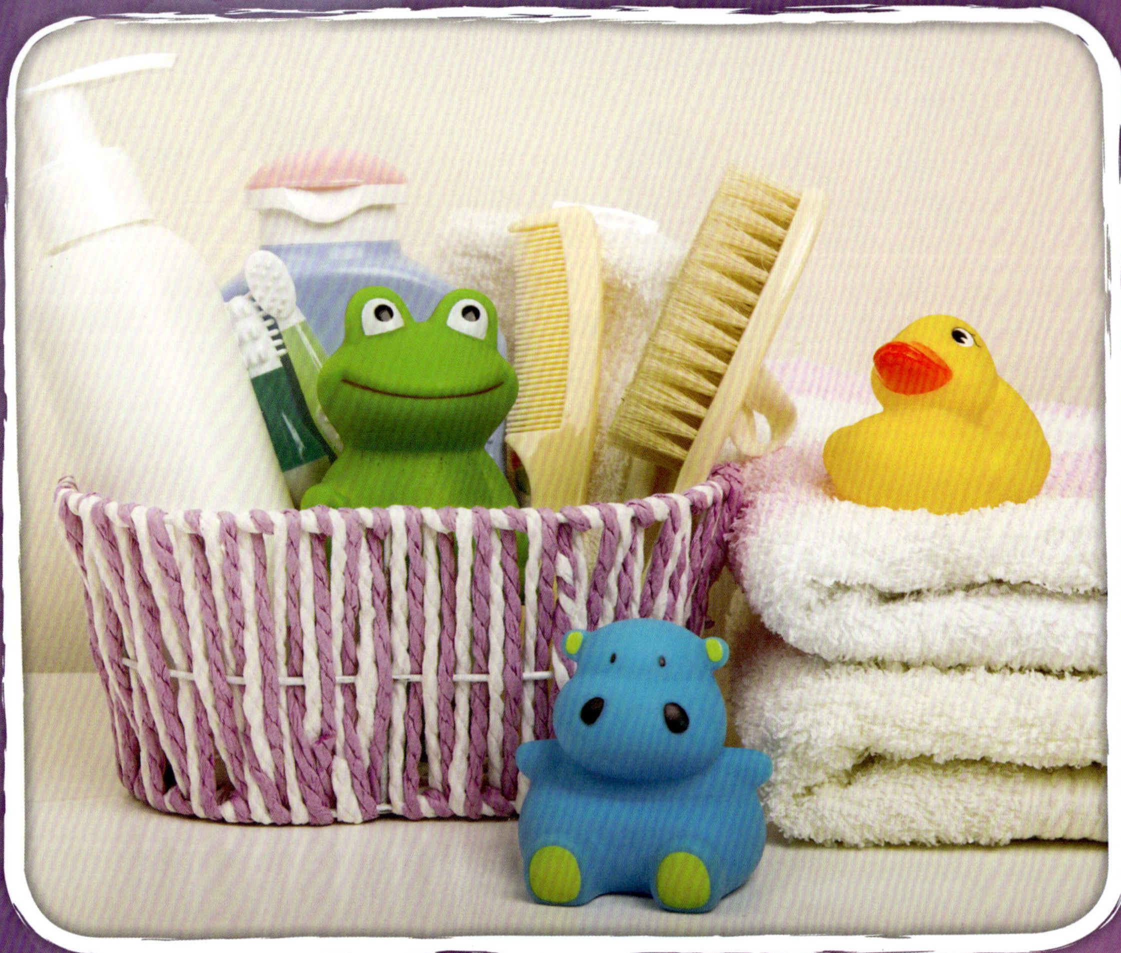

Go and find some

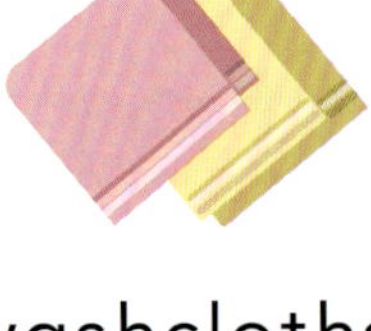 by the water.

washcloths

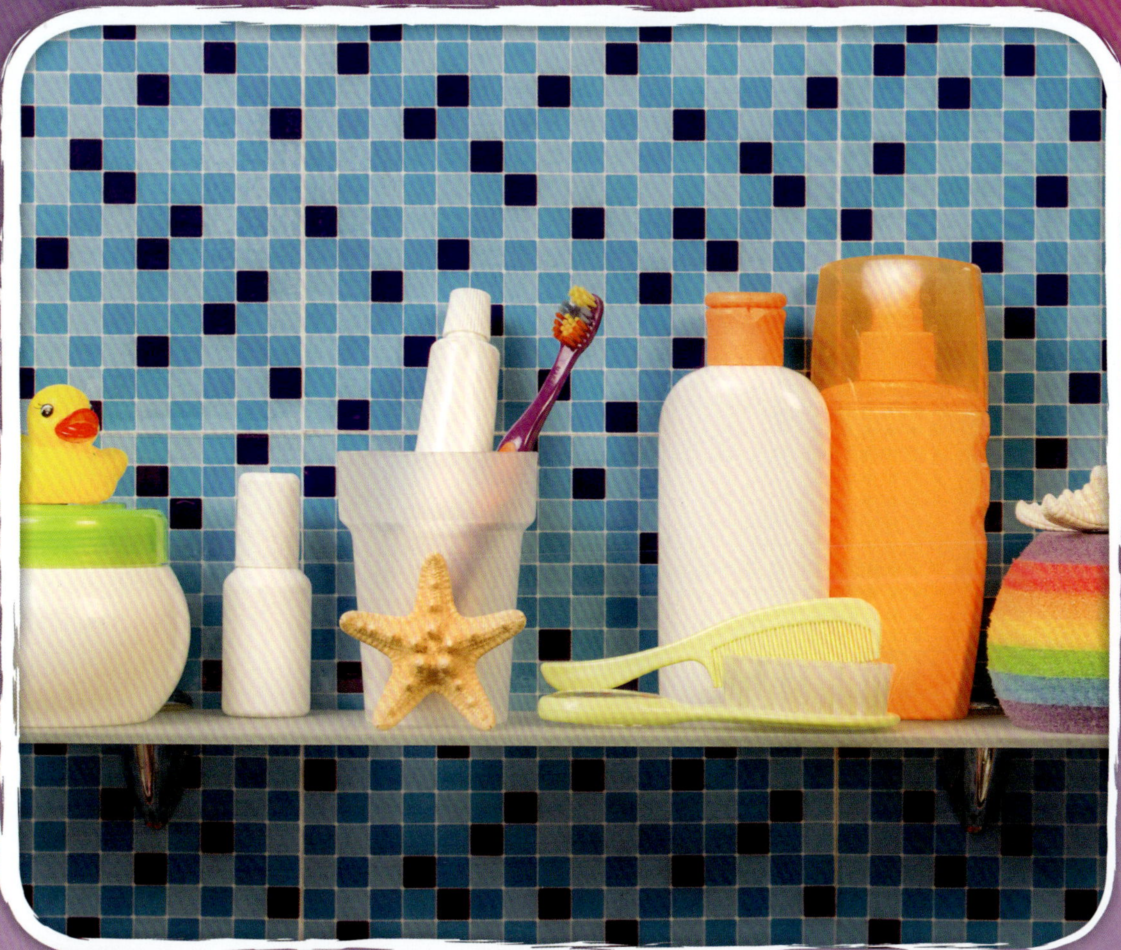

Go and find some

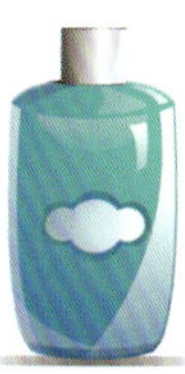

shampoo

by the water.

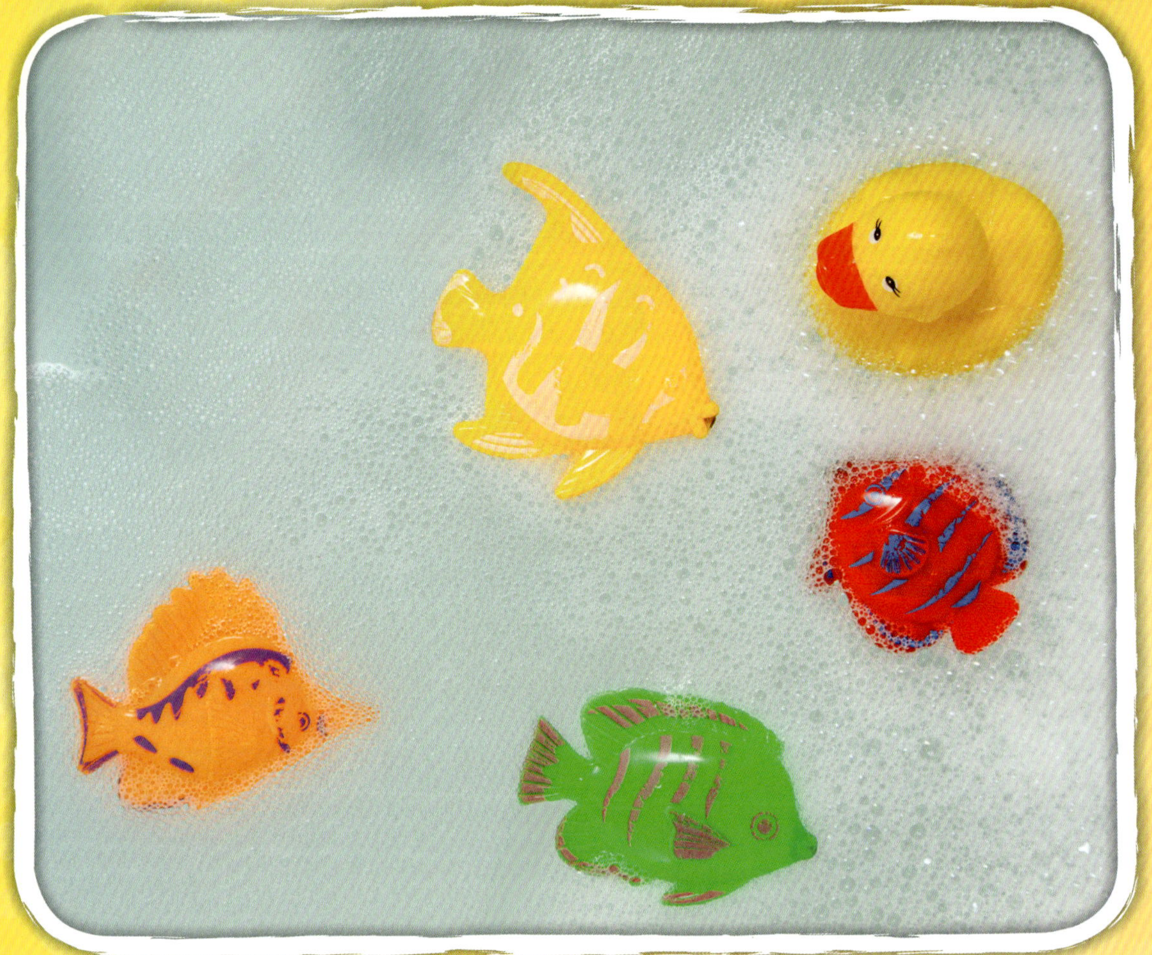

Go and find some

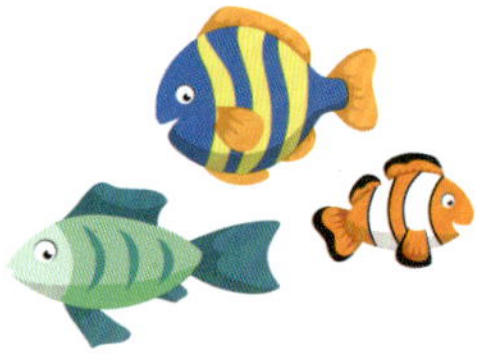 by the water.

fish

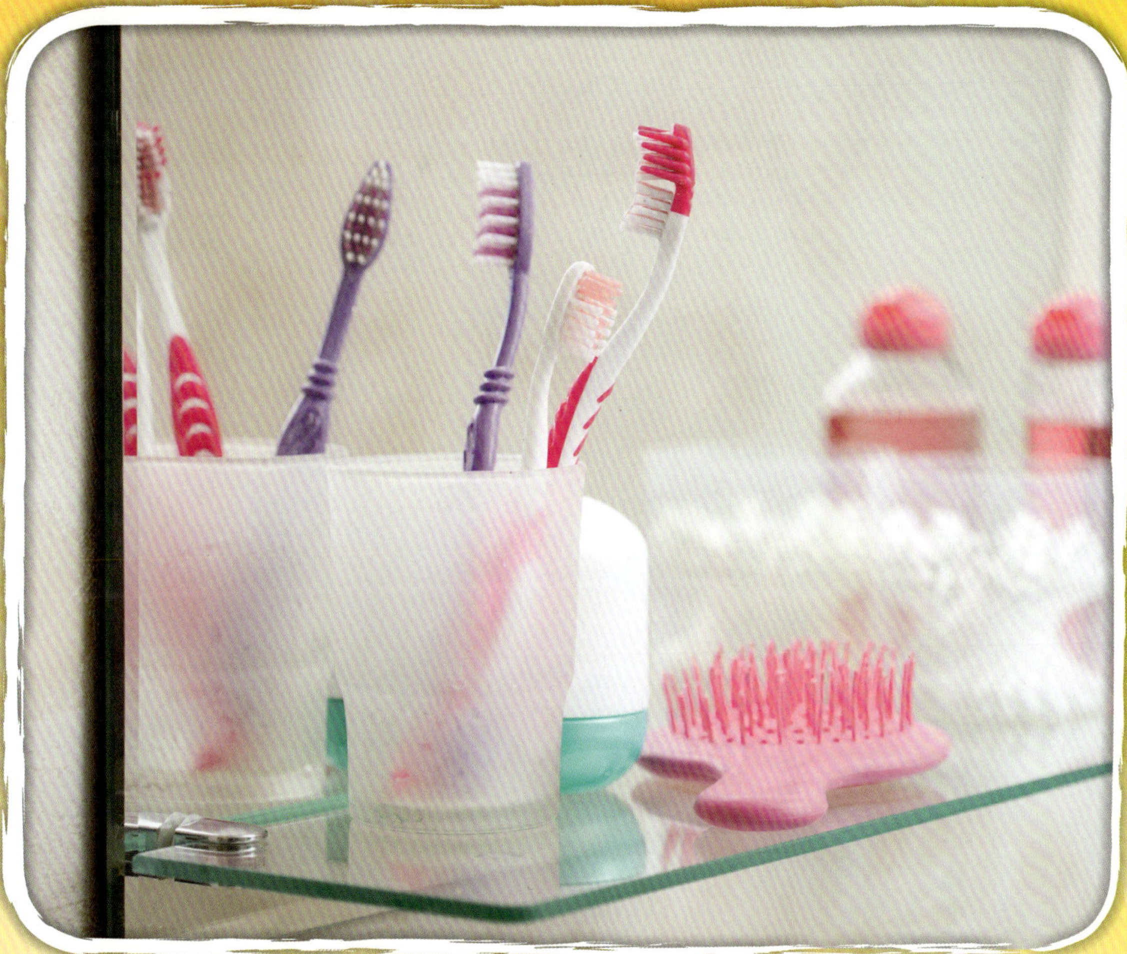

Go and find some

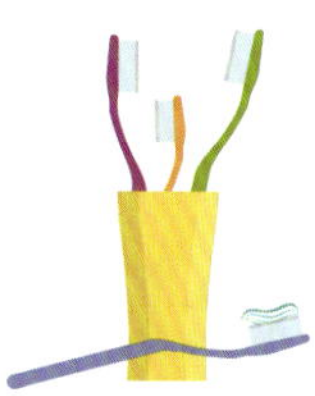 by the water.

toothbrushes

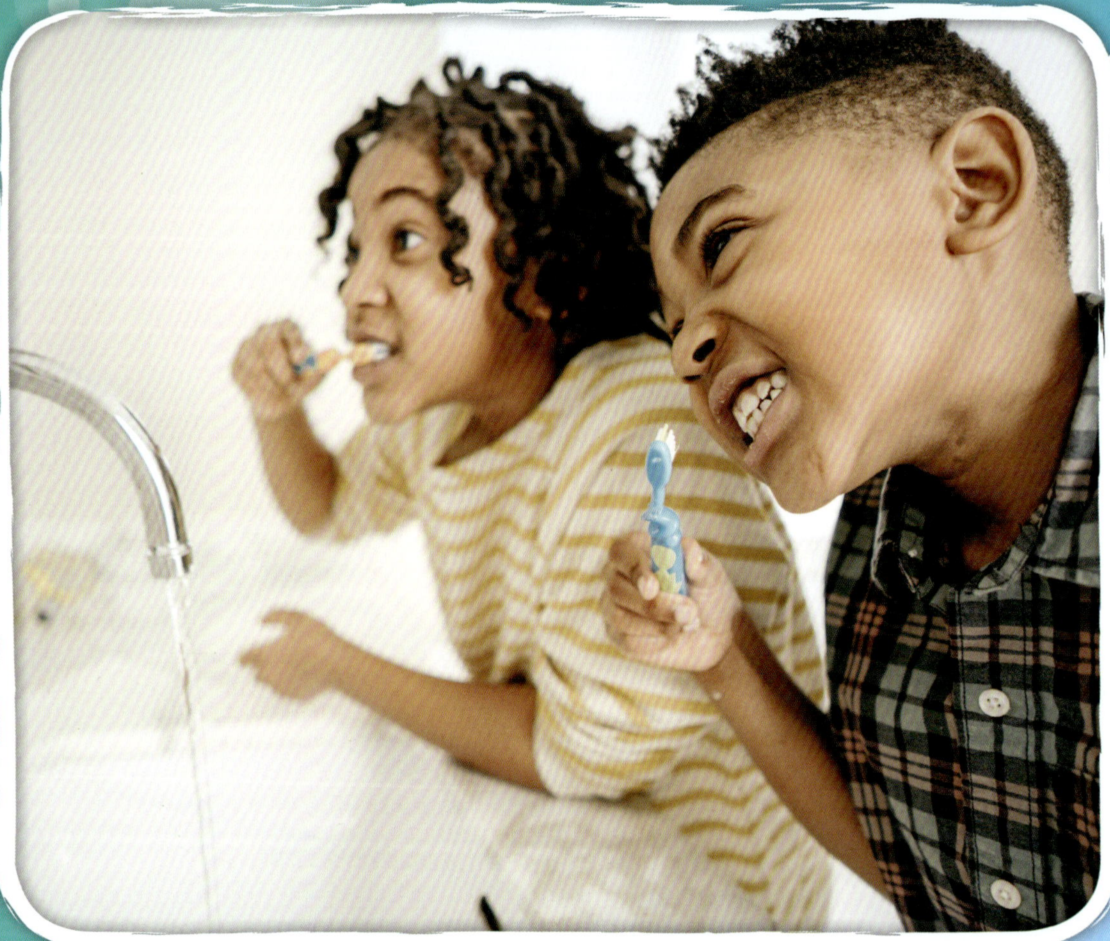

Go and find some

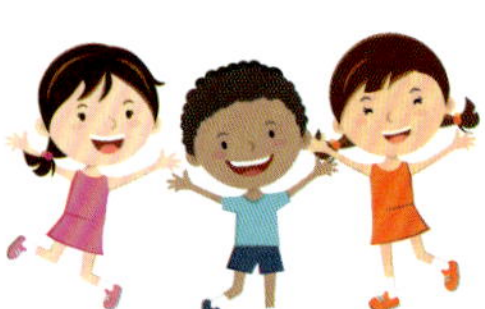 by the water.

kids

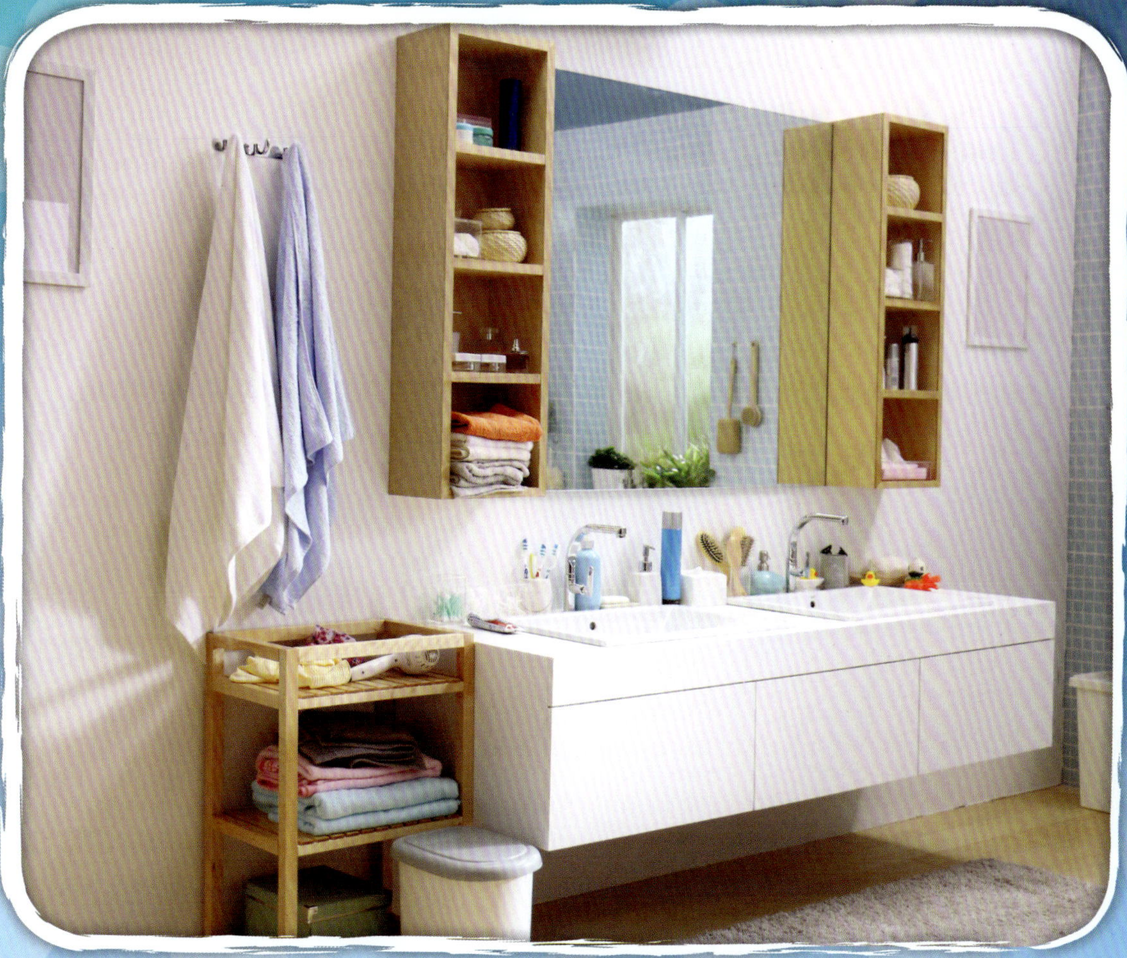

Go and find some

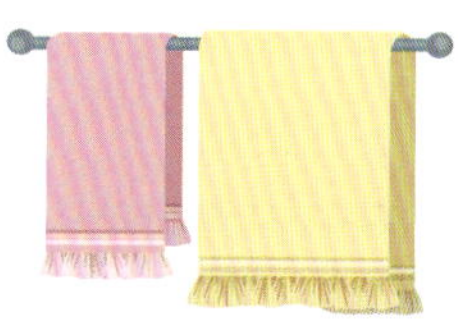 by the water.

towels

High-Frequency Words

New Words

by
find
go
some
water

Review Words

and
the